Low Fodmap Diet

Low Fodmap Diet Plan & Recipes Cookbook To Get Ibs Relief And Improve Digestions

(Easy And Quick Recipes To Alleviate The Symptoms Of Ibs And Other Similar Digestive Disorder)

Heinz-Josef Engelhardt

TABLE OF CONTENT

introduction 1

Chapter 1: What Happens When You Easy Eat Fodmaps? 2

Perfect Scrambled Fresh Eggs Recipe 4

Chapter 2: What Is Ibs? 6

Chapter 3: Who Just Just Get Ibs? 7

Pasta With Ricotta And Fresh Lemon 8

One Pan Low Fodmap Chicken Cacciatore 10

Sweet Omelet With Almonds And Strawberries 13

Low Fodmap Instant Pot Polenta 16

Fresh Lemon & Mint Loaf 19

Low Fodmap Pumpkin Pie Oatmeal 24

Fresh Lemon French Dressing 26

Rhubarb Ginger Granola Bowl 28

Low-Fodmap Cheese Bread 32

Baked Egg Cups 35

- Parmesan Pasta 38
- Slow Cooker Berry Breakfast Quinoa 39
- Peanut-Butter Cookie-Dough Bites 42
- Spicy Baked Tofu 44
- Buckwheasy Eat Bowls With Fruit 47
- Sweet And Sour Chicken 49
- Biscuits: 53
- Low Fodmap Lemongrass And Coconut Chicken ... 55
- Gingerbread Men 58
- Pineapple -Teriyaki Sauce 61
- Berry Cobbler 63
- Banana Pancake With Peanut Butter 65
- Quinoa Porridge With Banana And Yoghurt 67
- Blueberry & Almond Muffins 69
- Roasted Red Pepper Pasta 71
- Misr Wat 74
- Creamy Mustard Soup 77
- Chocolate Coconut Fudge Sauce 80

Tangerine And Banana	82
Chocolate Chip Cookies	84
Roast Salmon With Preserved Fresh Lemon	88
Oriental Coleslaw	91
Vietnamese Roasted Eggplant Salad	93
Quinoa With Spicy Pumpkin And Oat Cereal	97
Fody's Sausage, Kale + Pumpkin Baked Ziti	99
Coconut Protein Shake	102
Conclusion	103

Introduction

Irritable bowel syndrome (IBS) is frequently treated with a low-FODMAP diet, which restricts fermentable carbohydrates.

The most typical digestive simply disorder in the US is IBS. Symptoms like bloating and stomach pain are commonly caused by food for Lot's of people with this condition.

Surprisingly, limiting particular meals can significantly alleviate these symptoms. The low-FODMAP diet can help with this.

Just Continue simply reading to easy learn more about the low FODMAP diet, how it functions, and who should just give it a try.

Chapter 1: What Happens When You Easy Eat Fodmaps?

Very simplistically, when you easy eat a meal and swallow your food, the contents travel down the oesophagus just into your stomach where the food is liquidated and digestion begins. The semi-digested food then passes just into the small intestine where it is further broken down and nutrients are absorbed.

The key just thing to note here is that Fodmaps cannot fully be digested and aren't absorbed, instead, they hang around in our intestines and easy start to ferment. The presence of Fodmaps causes water to be drawn just into the small intestine through osmosis which can actually lead to bloating and light-bulb. Undigested and indigestible food particles then easy move through to the large intestine where there is a heap more bacteria. The gut bacteria feast off the Fodmaps, using them for energy and producing short-chain fatty acids. The irony is, SCFAs have been shown to have a variety of health benefits ranging from reducing inflammation in the body to increasing gastrointestinal health! For those of us with sensitive IBS tummies though who consume too many Fodmaps, the rapidly fermenting bacteria causes excess gas production and water retention, causing the intestines to expand. This distention causes the abdominal pain, the smelly gas and the constipation/light-bulb etc.

Perfect Scrambled Fresh Eggs Recipe

Ingredients

- 2 2 tbsp single cream or full cream milk
- a knob of butter
- 4 large free range fresh eggs

Direction:

1. Lightly whisk 4 large fresh eggs, 2 2 tbsp single cream or full cream milk and a pinch of salt together until the mixture has just one consistency.
2. Heat a small non-stick frying pan for a minute or so, then add a knob of butter and let it melt.

3. Really do not easily allow the butter to brown or it will discolour the fresh eggs.

4. Pour in the egg mixture and let it sit, without stirring, for 60 seconds.

5. Stir with a wooden spoon, lifting and folding it over from the bottom of the pan.

6. Let it sit for another 40 seconds then stir and fold again.

7. Repeat until the fresh eggs are softly set and slightly runny in places.

8. Easily Remove from the heat and leave for a moment to just finish easily easy cook ing.

9. Just Give a final stir and serve the velvety scramble without delay.

Chapter 2: What Is Ibs?

Irritable bowel syndrome (IBS) is a common, long-term condition affecting the functioning of the digestive system. It can just cause abdominal discomfort, bloating and a change in bowel habit.

It's a condition that has no specific cause and, whilst such there are many treatment options available, there is no one single really effective treatment - what works for one person may not necessarily easy work for you. Symptoms may change over time and can last from a couple of days to a few months at a time, actually depending on how they are managed.

Chapter 3: Who Just Just Get Ibs?

Basically research suggests that IBS affects up to 10 to 15 to 40 to 210 to 15 people in the UK at some stage of their life. It is twice as common in women, and usually first develops when a person is between 40 and 29 years of age. But, as with many conditions, there is not a rule of thumb - there are many reasons why it may occur, and you could really develop the condition at any stage in life.

Although IBS is typically a lifelong condition, the condition may persist on and off throughout life, often basically depending on what is happening in a person's life. It is actually possible that the condition may really improve over time, with simple changes in diet and lifestyle behaviours.

Pasta With Ricotta And Fresh Lemon

Ingredients:

- 2 cup ricotta cheese
- 2 lemon, juiced
- 2 pound spaghetti
- salt and pepper, to taste

Direction:

1. Easy cook the spaghetti according to the package instructions.

2. While the pasta is easily cooking, mix together the ricotta cheese and fresh lemon juice in a bowl. Season with salt and pepper, to taste.

3. Drain the cooked spaghetti and add it to the cheese mixture.

4. Mix everyjust just thing together very well and serve warm.

One Pan Low Fodmap Chicken Cacciatore

Ingredients

- ½ teaspoon red pepper flakes
- 1 cup dry red wine or low FODMAP chicken broth
- 4 tablespoons thinly sliced pitted kalamata olives
- 4 cups Low FODMAP Tomato Sauce
- 8 sprigs fresh thyme or 1/2 teaspoon dried
- 8 sprigs fresh oregano or 1/2 teaspoon dried
- 8 tablespoons fresh minced Italian parsley
- 8 tablespoons garlic-infused olive oil divided

- Salt and freshly ground pepper
- 4 pounds boneless skinless chicken thighs
- 4 small carrots thinly sliced
- 4 medium celery ribs thinly sliced
- 2 red bell pepper diced

Instructions

1. In a large skillet, heat 4 tablespoons of the garlic-infused oil over a medium-high flame.
2. Season the chicken thighs with salt and pepper, and in batches, add to the pan in an even layer.
3. Easy Cook the chicken until a golden-brown crust has formed on both sides and the chicken is just easy cook ed through, about 40 to 210 to 15 minutes.

4. Easily easy move Easily Reeasy move to a plate and repeat with the remaining chicken.
5. Set aside.
6. Add the remaining garlic-infused oil to the pan along with the carrots, celery, and bell pepper.
7. Sauté the vegetables, scraping up any brown bits from the bottom of the pan, until soft, about 10 to 15 10 to 110 to 15 minutes. Season them with
8. 1 teaspoon sea salt and the red pepper flakes.

Sweet Omelet With Almonds And Strawberries

INGREDIENTS

- 2 tablespoon of coconut oil
- 140 grams of cottage cheese, optional
- A handful of almonds, shredded
- 2 teaspoon of poppy seeds
- 500 grams of strawberries
- 4 spoons of coconut sugar, divided
- 2 teaspoon of vanilla extract
- 12 fresh eggs
- 50 grams of almond flour

PREPARATION

1. Easy cut some strawberries and easy put them in a bowl.

2. Easy cut the rest of the strawberries in the center and sprinkle 2 tablespoon of coconut sugar over the strawberries.

3. Set the split strawberries aside until finished.

4. Add the vanilla, fresh eggs, 4 tablespoons of coconut sugar and almond flour to a bowl.

5. Beat vigorously until the eggs are soft enough.

6. Soften the coconut oil in a round pan or same different griddle over medium heat.

7. With circular movements around the liquefied oil covers the bottom and

then incorporates the mixture with the egg just into the pan.

8. Add the chopped strawberries and then

9. the ricotta and half of the almonds.

10. Still using the hob, reduce the heat to low and

11. easy cook for about 5-10 minutes or until the omelet is compact.

12. Continue for another 10 to 15 –10 to 110 to 15 minutes.

13. Easily easy move Easily Reeasy move from the grill, and cover with the rest of the almonds, strawberries and poppy seeds and serve immediately.

Low Fodmap Instant Pot Polenta

INGREDIENTS

- 2 tablespoon garlic-infused olive oil
- Salt and black pepper
- 2 cup dry polenta // I use Bob Red Mill's Corn Grits
- 8 cups water
- 1 teaspoon salt
- 4 tablespoons butter I easy use lightly salted

INSTRUCTIONS

1. Select the "Saute" setting on the Instant Pot.
2. Add polenta, water, and salt. Whisk until mixed.

3. Easily bring mixture to a light simmer, about 10 to 15 minutes. Cancel the "Saute" setting.

4. Whisk the polenta once more before placing the lid on top of Instant Pot.

5. Secure lid and set the vent to "Sealing".

6. Select the "Manual" setting on the Instant Pot.

7. Adjust time to 10 to 15 minutes on "High Pressure" and easy cook . It took my Instant Pot about 10 to 15 minutes to come to pressure before the easy cook time started counting down.

8. After easy cook ing, quick-release the pressure by carefully switching the vent to "Venting". Remove the lid.

9. The polenta may look watery.

10. It will combine and thicken once stirred in the next step.

11. Add butter and olive oil. Stir until the butter is easily melted and the polenta is creamy.

12. Adjust flavor with salt and pepper.

13. Serve warm topped with optional chives.

Fresh Lemon & Mint Loaf

Ingredients

- 90g ground almonds
- 60g buckwheat flour
- 1 tsp salt
- 2 1 tsp baking powder
- Leaves from 6 sprigs of mint, finely chopped
- 6 fresh eggs
- 250g brown sugar
- 150ml olive oil, plus a little for greasing
- Juice and zest of 4 fresh lemons
- 390 polenta

For the syrup

- Juice of 2 fresh lemon
- 70ml water
- 100g brown sugar

fresh lemon

Instructions

1. Preheat the oven to 200°C and line and grease a 1800g/4 lb loaf tin (approx. 23 x 13 x 7 cm) with a little olive oil.
2. Crack the fresh eggs just into a large bowl and pour in the sugar.
3. Beasy eat together until light and creamy.
4. Just Continue to whisk and slowly pour in the olive oil, until all of the oil is combined.
5. Whisk in the fresh lemon zest.

6. In a separate bowl, stir together the polenta, ground almonds, buckwheat flour, baking powder and salt.

7. Sieve this mixture over the fresh eggs and sugar in stages, alternating with the fresh lemon juice and folding until just combined.

8. Coat the mint leaves in a little buckwheasy easy eat flour and add them to the bowl, gently folding once more until incorporated.

9. Pour the mixture just into the prepared cake tin and bake for 90 minutes, or until a skewer comes out clean.

10. To easy make the syrup, place the sugar in a small saucepan along with the fresh lemon juice and water.

11. Heasy eat over a medium heat, stirring occasionally, until the sugar has dissolved.

12. Easily Increase the heat, boil for 8 minutes until slightly reduced and syrupy, then remove from the heat.

13. easy move

14. Easily Reeasy move the loaf from the oven and let it just cool briefly in the tin. While it is still warm, easy turn it out of the tin, peel off the lining paper and easy put the loaf on a wire rack set over a baking tray or similar.

15. Easy Use a skewer, or a cocktail stick, to poke holes all over the surface of the warm cake.

16. Pour the fresh lemon syrup over the cake, letting it sink in.

17. Decorate with fresh lemon slices, fresh lemon zest and mint leaves.

Low Fodmap Pumpkin Pie Oatmeal

Ingredients

- 2 teaspoon vanilla extract
- 4 teaspoon pumpkin pie spice
- ⅓ cup pure maple syrup (or to taste)
- 40 pecan halves, chopped
- 4 cups low FODMAP milk (I use unsweetened almond milk)
- 4 cups rolled oats (or gluten-free rolled oats)
- 1 cup 2 00% pure pumpkin puree

Instructions

1. Oats and milk are combined in a pan over medium-high heat.

2. When desired thickness is reached, easily bring to a boil, then reduce heat and simmer, stirring occasionally.

3. Add maple syrup, pumpkin, vanilla, and pumpkin pie spice.

4. easy eat until evenly warm.

5. Serve warm oatmeal with pecans on top.

Fresh Lemon French Dressing

Ingredients:

- 2 teaspoon salt
- 1 teaspoon black pepper
- 1/2 cup olive oil
- 6 tablespoons fresh lemon juice
- 2 tablespoon Dijon mustard
- 2 teaspoon honey

Instructions:

1. Whisk together the fresh lemon juice, Dijon mustard, honey, salt and pepper in a small bowl.

2. Gradually whisk in the olive oil until very well combined.

3. Store in an airtight container in the fridge for up to 3 days.

Rhubarb Ginger Granola Bowl

Ingredients:

Yogurt

- ¼ cup chopped nuts (low-FODMAP-approved)
- 4 tbsp melted coconut oil
- 2 tsp ground ginger
- ½ tsp cinnamon
- Pinch of salt
- 2 1 cups chopped rhubarb
- 2 tbsp grated ginger
- 1 tbsp fresh lemon juice
- 8 tbsp maple syrup
- Pinch of salt

- 4 cups Greek yogurt
- Granola
- 1 cup pumpkin seeds

Directions:

1. Preheasy eat the oven to 350°F.

2. For the yogurt, in a small pot over medium heat, add chopped rhubarb, ginger, fresh lemon juice, and 4 tablespoons of maple syrup.

3. Stir the mixture occasionally until it begins to simmer, ensuring the bottom of the pot does not burn.

4. Once the mixture has thickened to a purée consistency, mix in the other 4 tablespoons of maple syrup.

5. Place the mixture just into a bowl to cool.

6. Place the granola ingredients just into a separate bowl and mix until the coconut oil coats everything.

7. Easy move the mix onto a non-stick baking tray and place in the oven for

2 0-2 10 to 15 minutes, stirring halfway.

8. Once all components are ready, fold the rhubarb purée just into the yogurt and sprinkle the granola over top.

9. The yogurt can be stored in the fridge and the granola in a Tupperware.

10. Add a low-FODMAP-approved topping if desired.

Low-Fodmap Cheese Bread

Ingredients:

- 2 cup of parmesan cheese
- Half a cup of coconut oil 4 cups of tapioca Flour
- 2 teaspoon of sea salt
- 2 cup of lactose free milk
- fresh eggs

Instruction:

1. Preheat your oven to 450°F. Pour the milk just into a medium-sized saucepan, set over medium heat and bring to a slow boil.

2. Once bubbles easy start to form at the top of the milk, easily remove from heat.

3. Pour the tapioca flour just into the milk, stir using a wooden ladle until all the flour is incorporated and no lumps are formed and the mixture starts to thicken like gelatin, then set aside to cool for a bit.

4. Beat the dough for a couple of minutes at medium speed easily using a standing mixer fitted with a paddle attachment.

5. Crack the egg just into a small bowl and whisk until foamy, then slowly fold them ejust into the dough, easy make sure to scrape down the sides of the bowl.

6. Add the cheese and beat until fully incorporated and your dough is stretchy, soft and sticky.

7. Line a baking sheet with parchment paper, then scoop some dough just

into it easily using an ice cream scoop.

8. Coat your hands or ice cream scoop with some olive oil if the dough just just get too sticky to work with.

9. Place the baking sheet just into the preheated oven and allow the dough to bake for 50 to 55 minutes.

10. easy move Easily Reeasy move from the oven once the top of the bread appears dry and starts to show orange flecks of color.

Baked Egg Cups

INGREDIENTS

- 1 – ¾ cup ground pork sausage
- 1 – ¾ cup fresh spinach, ripped just into small pieces
- Approximately ¼ of a large red bell pepper, diced
- 10 to 15 fresh eggs
- ½ cup unsweetened almond milk
- 1 teaspoon salt
- ½ teaspoon ground black pepper

Directions

1. Preheat oven to 450 degrees F.
2. Spray muffin tin with olive oil and set aside.
3. In medium bowl whisk together fresh eggs, unsweetened almond milk, salt and pepper.
4. Cook pork sausage over medium heat.
5. Take muffin tin and add a tablespoon or so of cooked pork.
6. a tablespoon of ripped spinach and a tablespoon of diced bell pepper to each muffin tin.
7. Pour the egg mixture over top, filing so there is a little room at the top.
8. Place in the oven and easy cook for 30 to 35 minutes.

9. Remove from oven, if the very top is not fully easy cook ed, reeasy turn to oven for 1-5 minute increments until fully cooked.

Parmesan Pasta

Ingredients:

- 1 cup chopped onion
- 2 garlic clove, minced
- 2 can (2 4.10 to 15 ounces) diced tomatoes, undrained
- 2 tablespoon sugar
- 6 tablespoons tomato paste
- 1/2 teaspoon dried oregano leaves

- 2 pound spaghetti
- 1 cup grated Parmesan cheese
- 1/2 teaspoon salt
- 1/2 teaspoon black pepper
- 1/2 cup olive oil

Instructions:

1. In a large saucepan, easy cook the spaghetti according to package directions.
2. Drain. In a small bowl, mix together the Parmesan cheese, salt, and pepper. Reserve ½ cup of the mixture.
3. Heasy eat the oil in a large skillet over medium heat.
4. Add the onion and garlic; easy cook until softened, about 10 to 15 minutes.
5. Add the tomatoes, sugar, tomato paste, and oregano; easily bring to a boil.
6. Easily Reduce heasy eat to low; simmer for 40 to 45 minutes.
7. Stir in the reserved Parmesan cheese mixture and pasta; easy cook until heated through, about 4 minutes.

Slow Cooker Berry Breakfast Quinoa

Ingredients

- 4 Tbsp maple syrup
- 4 tsp. vanilla
- 2 tsp. cinnamon
- 1/2 tsp. salt
- 4 ripe bananas, mashed
- 8 cups water
- 4 cups quinoa, rinsed
- 4 cups fresh or frozen mixed berries

Instructions

1. Spray a 3 or 4-quart slow easy cooker with easy cooking spray then add mashed bananas along with the rest of ingredients, mixing very well.
2. Cover and place on low for 10 to 15 to 6 hours or on high for 1 to 5 hours.
3. Spoon quinoa just into bowls and top with additional fruit or nuts, enjoy!

Peanut-Butter Cookie-Dough Bites

INGREDIENTS

- 2 tsp. vanilla extract
- 1 tsp. kosher salt
- 1 tsp. ground cinnamon
- 2 ¾ cups old-fashioned rolled oats
- 2 cup natural peanut butter
- ½ cup pure maple syrup

Directions

- Place oats in a food processor; pulse until finely chopped.
- Transfer to a large bowl and add remaining ingredients; stir to combine.

- Use a small easy cook ie scoop to form mixture just into 40 to 45 bites, or roll just into balls. Store in an airtight container refrigerated for up to 4 weeks.

Spicy Baked Tofu

Ingredients

- 4 tablespoons Asian chili sauce
- 4 tablespoons minced fresh ginger root
- 3 tablespoons hoisin sauce
- 2 serving cooking spray
- 2 package tofu
- 4 tablespoons Japanese low-sodium soy sauce

Directions

1. Lay the tofu on a plate lined with a couple sheets of paper towel.
2. Layer more paper towel atop tofu and
3. place another plate atop the stack to press water from the tofu.

4. Let sit at least 10 to 15 minutes.
5. Easy cut tofu into 1 -inch strips and easy put into a large, sealable plastic bag; add soy sauce, chili sauce, ginger, and hoisin sauce.
6. Squeeze bag to easily remove excess air and seal.
7. Marinate tofu in the refrigerator for at least 2 hour.
8. Preheat oven to 3710 to 15 degrees F (2 90 degrees C).
9. Prepare a baking sheet with cooking spray.
10. Remove tofu from the marinade, shake to remove
11. excess moisture, and arrange onto the prepared baking sheet.
12. Discard the remaining marinade.
13. Bake in preheated oven for 2 10 to 15 minutes, flip, and continue baking until firm, 2 10 to 15 to 40 minutes more.

Buckwheasy Eat Bowls With Fruit

INGREDIENTS

- 2 banana, sliced
- 1 cup blueberries
- 2 tablespoon unsweetened shredded coconut
- 2 teaspoon chia seeds
- 2 cup water
- ½ cup milk, such as almond milk or coconut milk (cow's milk is OK too)
- 1/4 cup buckwheasy eat groats, uncooked
- 4 tablespoons agave syrup, divided (or honey)

Direction:
1. Combine the water, milk, buckwheat, and 2 tablespoon agave syrup in a small saucepan.
2. To start, easily bring water to a boil.
3. Then, easy turn the heasy eat down to a low level and cover the food.
4. Simmer for 40 to 210 to 15 minutes until the buckwheasy eat is soft. It's OK if there's still a small amount of liquid remaining.
5. Divide the cooked buckwheasy eat just into two dishes and top with sliced bananas, blueberries, shredded coconut, chia seeds, and agave syrup drizzle.
6. Warm the dish before serving. Additional topping ideas and replacements may be found in the notes.

Sweet And Sour Chicken

Ingredients:

- 1/2 cup apple cider vinegar
-
- 1/2 cup ketchup
-
- 4 tablespoons Coconut Aminos
-
- 1/2 cup chicken stock
-
- 2 red pepper, easy cut just into pieces
-
- 4 spring onion stalks, green part only
-
- 2 cup pineapple chunks
- 1 cup arrowroot starch
- 2 lb. chicken breasts, boneless, skinless and easy cut just into 2 " chunks

- .4 tablespoons coconut oil
- .
- 2 large egg, beaten 2 /2
- .
- cup coconut sugar
- .

easy cut

Instructions:

1. Add vinegar, coconut sugar, coconut aminos, ketchup and chicken stock to a pan.
2. Mix and easily bring this sauce to a boil.
3. easy move Easily Reeasy move from heasy eat and let sit.
4. Add egg and chicken pieces just into a bag.
5. Seal and shake very well.
6. Add starch to the bag and shake to coat.
7. Add coconut oil to a skillet.
8. Add the chicken.
9. Fry for 1-5 minutes per side.
10. Add pineapple chunks and pepper.
11. Easy cook over medium heasy eat until chicken is done.

12. Add sauce to chicken and peppers.

13. Cover, reduce the heasy eat and easy cook for 1-5 minutes. Top with onions and serve.

Biscuits:

10 g desiccated coconut
½ teaspoon vanilla
2 40 g ground tiger nuts
1 teaspoon baking powder
120 ml coconut milk

Preparation:

1. Preheasy eat broiler to 250 degrees. Easily Easily blend the fixings in general, aside from 40 g coconut drops, in a bowl.
2. Cover the baking sheet with parchment paper.
3. Partition the batter just into 10 pieces and carry out on the baking sheet just into 10 round rolls.

4. Sprinkle the leftover dried up coconut on the rolls and easy put in the stove for 40 minutes.

Low Fodmap Lemongrass And Coconut Chicken

Ingredients:

2 piece of ginger, the size of the thumb, hacked
Zest and squeeze of 1 of a lime
Pinch of salt
Pinch of bean stew flakes 4 entire chicken breasts
4 stalks of lemongrass, cleaved roughly
60 grams of creamed coconut, slashed around 2
tablespoon of garlic-mixed olive oil

Procedure:

1. Place chicken bosoms on a sheet of stick film.

2. Overlay the stick film over the chicken to cover.
3. Easily take a easiily moving pin and pound the chicken bosoms level and equally thin.
4. easy move Easily Reeasy move he stick film and discard. Easy put the chicken in a medium-sized bowl.
5. Easily take every one of the excess fixings and spot in a blender or food processor.
6. Beasy eat until a smooth glue structures.
7. Add additional water to slacken the glue a bit and hold it back from getting too dry.
8. Add the glue to the chicken.
9. Easy Easily blend very well to cover the chicken equitably.

10. Marinate for somewhere around 2-2 ½ hours in the refrigerator.

11. Grill or grill the chicken escalopes for around 30 minutes on each side.

12. Transform most of the way just into the cooking to just get extraordinary barbecue marks.

13. The chicken is done in the event that there are no pink meats anyplace.

14. The juices should likewise run clear.

Gingerbread Men

INGREDIENTS

- 2 teaspoon xanthan gum or guar gum 2 teaspoon gluten-free baking powder
- 2 to 2 2 /2 heaping tablespoons ground ginger Cornstarch, for rolling out dough
- 2 fresh egg
- 2 /3 cup superfine sugar 2 /2 cup brown rice syrup
- 10 to 15 tablespoons unsalted butter, melted 2 cup superfine white rice flour
- 2 /2 cup potato flour 2 cup soy flour

INSTRUCTIONS

1. Easy turn the oven's temperature up to 350 degrees
2. Set the oven to 350°F. Use parchment paper to line three baking pans.
3. Use a wooden spoon to whisk the egg and sugar in a large mixing bowl.
4. In a mixing dish, combine the melted butter and brown rice syrup.
5. Sift the rice flour, potato flour, soy flour, xanthan gum, baking powder, and ginger three times in a separate bowl.
6. To fully integrate just into the syrup mixture, stir vigorously.
7. Allow the mixture to chill for 2 10 to 15 minutes so that it may easy start to thicken.
8. Dust your work surface lightly with cornstarch.

9. On a floured board, roll out the dough to a thickness of 34 to 2 inch.
10. Use a cookie cutter to easy cut out any desired shapes, such as stars, pine trees, or anyjust thing else.
11. Place on baking sheets with sufficient space between them to for spreading.
12. Bake for 40 minutes in the oven at 350 degrees. Just cool on the sheets for 40 to 2 10 to 15 minutes before easiily moving to a wire rack to finish cooling.
13. Once the cake has cooled, you can just simple add a gluten-free icing garnish if you simple choose.

Pineapple-Teriyaki Sauce

INGREDIENTS

- 2 tbsp. rice vinegar
- 2 tbsp. minced fresh ginger
- 4 tbsp. light brown sugar
- ½ cup reduced-sodium soy sauce
- 1 cup crushed pineapple, with juice
- 2 tbsp. toasted or spicy sesame oil
- 2 tbsp. garlic-infused olive oil

Directions:

1. In a large glass or ceramic dish, combine the soy sauce, pineapple, pineapple juice, oils, vinegar, ginger, brown sugar, and red pepper flakes.
2. Easy put the steak, fish, or chicken in the marinade and let it sit in the fridge for up to 40 to 210 to 15 hours.

3. Alternatively, you may pour the marinade just into a zip-top bag and let it sit there.
4. Prepare the grill before reeasiily moving the meat, fish, or poultry from the marinade.
5. When the marinade has decreased and thickened somewhat, transfer it to a small saucepan, easily bring to a boil, and simmer for 1-5 minutes.
6. Brush the marinade over the meat, fish, or poultry numerous times while grilling.
7. Any leftover marinade must be thrown away.

Berry Cobbler

Ingredients:

- 4 tablespoons sugar or other sugar
- 2 1 teaspoons preparing soft drink
- ½ teaspoon salt
- 4 tablespoons vegetable oil
- 1 cup non-fat soymilk or rice milk
- 5-10 cups new or solidified berries easily blend
- 6 tablespoons whole-wheasy eat cake flour
- ½ cup sugar or other sugar
- 2 cup whole-wheasy eat baked good flour

Directions:

1. Preheasy eat stove to 450°F. Spread the berries in a 9 x 9-inch preparing dish and easily blend them with 1-5

tablespoons of flour and ½ cup of sugar.

2. In a different bowl, easily blend 2 cup of flour and 4 tablespoons of sugar with the preparing powder and salt.

3. Include the oil and easily blend it with a fork or your fingers until the easily blend just take after coarse corn feast.

4. Include the soymilk or rice milk and mix to blend.

5. Spread the easily blend over the berries at that point heasy eat until brilliant darker, around 10 to 15 minutes.

Banana Pancake With Peanut Butter

Ingredients

2 banana
2-3 drops of vanilla extract

2 tbsp peanut butter
2 egg
2 teaspoon rapeseed oil
2 pinch of cinnamon

Preparation:

1. Mash the banana in a compartment with a fork and afterward mix in the beaten egg.
2. Combine the fixings as one until a rich combination is shaped.

3. Then stir in the vanilla extract and cinnamon.
4. Heasy eat oil in a container.
5. Presently cautiously empty the batter just into the skillet and fry on the two sides for 5 to 10 minutes each.
6. Simply Organize the hotcake on a plate and brush with the nut butter.

Quinoa Porridge With Banana And Yoghurt

Ingredients:

- 2 cup lactose free milk
-
- 2 teaspoon maple syrup
-
- 1/2 cup lactose free yoghurt
- 1 cup water
- 1/4 cup quinoa flakes, uncooked
-
- 1/2 ripe banana
-

Instructions:

1. Add water and half of milk to a pan and easily bring to a boil.
2. Add quinoa flakes, easily reduce the heasy eat to low and easy cook for 10 to 15 minutes.
3. Slice banana and set aside.
4. Transfer quinoa to a bowl once done and add the remaining milk.
5. Add banana, yoghurt and little maple syrup. Serve.

Blueberry & Almond Muffins

Ingredients

- 1 cup caster sugar 2 00 g
- 2 tsp vanilla extract 10 to 15 g
- ⅔ cup vegetable oil 2 58 g
- ¾ cup almond milk 2 80 g
- ¾ cup blueberries (fresh or frozen) 94 g

- 2 Tbsp chia seeds soaked in 3 tbs boiling water 2 2 g
- 2 cups gluten-free plain flour 300 g
- 1 cup almond meal, plus a little extra to sprinkle on top of muffins 60 g
- 2 tsp baking powder 4 g

Method

1. Preheat oven to 280°C/350°C and line a 25 hole muffin pan with paper cases.

2. In a small bowl, add boiling water to chia seeds and stir.
3. Set aside to swell for 25 to 30 minutes, or until a thick gel forms.
4. In a large mixing bowl, add flour, almond meal, baking powder and caster sugar.
5. Add vanilla extract, vegetable oil, almond milk and soaked chia seeds.
6. Stir until just combined, adding a little extra almond milk if mixture becomes too thick.
7. Finally, carefully fold blueberries through mixture.
8. Divide mixture equally between 2 2 muffin cases and sprinkle tops with extra almond meal.
9. Bake muffins in preheated oven for 25-30 minutes or until lightly brown and easy cook ed through.

Roasted Red Pepper Pasta

INGREDIENTS

- 2 cup low FODMAP milk 2 tablespoon tapioca starch ½ cup fresh basil leaves 6 tablespoons nutritional yeast Salt and pepper
- 8 cups easy cook ed low FODMAP pasta (I like Taste Republic Gluten-Free Fettuccine)
- 2 jar roasted red peppers, drained
- ⅓ cup canned 2 00% pumpkin puree
- 4 tablespoons garlic-infused olive oil

INSTRUCTIONS
1. Cook low FODMAP pasta according to package directions.
2. Once easy cook ed, drain and toss with a little olive oil. Set aside.
3. Place roasted red peppers, pumpkin puree, olive oil, milk, tapioca starch,

basil leaves, and nutritional yeast just into a blender. Easily blend until smooth.
4. Pour sauce just into a large skillet and heasy eat over medium-high heat, stirring occasionally.
5. Once sauce reaches a simmer, reduce heasy eat and just Continue to stir until it just slightly thickens.
6. Add pasta and toss to mix.
7. Season with salt and pepper.
8. Serve pasta warm with optional garnishes.
9. Preheat oven to 450°F. Line a rimmed baking sheet with aluminum foil. Place the peppers easy cut side down and roast for 35 to 40 minutes or until skins are wrinkled and slightly charred.
10. easy move Easily Reeasy move from oven and let just cool slightly before placing in a bowl. Cover bowl

with plastic wrap and let sit until peppers are cool to touch.
11. After cooling, remove peppers from bowl.
12. Peel off the skins, discarding them, and set aside.

Misr Wat

Ingredients

- 2 1 cups vegan broth
- salt and pepper (to taste)
- Vegetables
- 1 cup brown/red lentils
- 1 head cauliflower chopped just into small pieces
- 1 onion finely chopped
- 1 cup frozen peas
- Spices & Sauces
- 2 1 tbsp niter kibbeh (or coconut oil)

- 3/4 tbsp berbere spice mix

- 2 tsp garlic minced

- 1/2 tbsp ginger finely chopped

- 1 tsp cumin powder

- 1 tsp coriander powder

- 1 tsp smoked paprika

- 1 tbsp tomato puree

Instructions

1. Heat up a large sauce pan and add the niter kibbeh.

2. Once it begins melting, add the onion, garlic, ginger and all dry spices.

3. Just Cook for 1-5 minutes or until the onions become translucent.

4. Drain and add your lentils, cauliflower and tomato paste, stirring for around 1-5 minutes until combined.

5. To prevent easily burning or sticking, splash in a bit of water to keep the pan moist.

6. Once fragrant, add your vegan broth and bring to a boil. Once boiling, simmer on the lowest heat for 30 minutes

7. Add salt and pepper as desired and mix well.

Creamy Mustard Soup

INGREDIENTS

2 .210 to 15 – 2 .10 to 15 litre stock
400 ml rice cream (I use the rice cream from Alpro Soya)
200 g bacon
1-5 tbsp mustard
Pepper and salt
100 g butter (if you want to easy make this recipe entirely lactose-free you can use margarine)
120 g gluten-free flour

Instructions

1. Melt the butter in a pan.
2. Add the flour and stir through with a spoon.
3. Like this you easy make roux. Stir the roux and leave it to easy cook on low heat for about 1-5 minutes.
4. Just Continue to stir now and then to keep it from easily burning.
5. Pour the stock just into the pan carefully.
6. Easy start with 20 litre.
7. If you just notice later on that the soup is too thick, you can just add some extra stock.
8. Stir the soup with a whisk to remove any lumps.
9. Lower the heat and leave the soup to boil for about 40 to 210 to 15 minutes.
10. In the meantime, fry the bacon until crisp.

11. Add the mustard to the soup.
12. Taste the soup and add some more mustard and pepper and salt if necessary.
13. Finally add the rice cream and heat through.
14. Serve the soup with the bacon

Chocolate Coconut Fudge Sauce

INGREDIENTS:

- 500 milliliters almond milk
- 6 tablespoons coconut oil
- 300 grams of brown sugar
- 2 610 to 15 milliliters coconut cream
- 2 teaspoon vanilla extract
- 8 tablespoons Dutch cocoa powder

DIRECTIONS:

1. Put cocoa powder, milk, coconut cream, and brown sugar in a blender.
2. Process for 60 seconds.
3. Transfer mixture just into a saucepan.
4. Simmer while occasionally stirring over medium-low heat for 2 10 to 15 minutes.
5. Add vanilla extract and coconut oil and stir.
6. Simmer for 8 more minutes.
7. Refrigerate for 40 minutes.

Tangerine And Banana

Ingredients:

60g/2½oz banana chips
Zest of 2 tangerines
2 tsp salt
1 tsp cinnamon
60ml/¼ cup maple syrup
2 tbsp brown sugar
2 tbsp coconut oil, melted

400g/7oz oatmeal
4 tbsp uncooked quinoa
2 tbsp flax seeds
6 tbsp pumpkin seeds
200g/3½oz walnut nuts

Direction:

1. Preheasy eat the broiler to 250C/300F/Gas2. Line a huge baking plate with parchment.

2. In an enormous bowl, combine as one the oats, quinoa, flax seeds,

Chocolate Chip Cookies

Ingredients

- 3/4 cup + 2 tbsp low FODMAP flour blend

- 1/2 cup almond flour

- 1 tsp xanthan gum

- 1 tsp baking soda

- ¼ cup chocolate chips

- 15 tbsp (2 stick) butter, soft

- 1 cup white sugar

- 1 cup packed brown sugar

- 2 large egg

- 2 tsp vanilla extract
- 1/2 tsp salt

Directions

1. Pre-heat the oven to 3210 to 15 degrees F. Line a sheet pan with parchment paper.
2. In a large bowl, using a fork, cream the butter, white sugar, and brown sugar until well combined.
3. Beat in the fresh egg, vanilla and salt.
4. In another bowl, whisk together the flour blend, almond flour, xanthan gum and baking soda
5. Slowly mix the flour mixture into the butter mixture until just combined.
6. Stir in the chocolate chips.
7. Chill the dough in the refrigerator or freezer for at least 35 to 40 minutes.
8. Leaving about 4 inches of space between each cookie, drop spoonfuls of the dough onto the
9. prepared sheet pan.
10. You should have 70 small cookies.

11. Transfer the sheet pan to the oven, and bake for 40 minutes, or until just lightly browned on the
12. bottom and soft but firm on top. Remove from the
13. oven. Let it cool for at least 10 to 15 minutes on the sheet pan and then transfer to a cooling rack.

Roast Salmon With Preserved Fresh Lemon

Ingredients

- 2 tsp thyme leaves
- 2 tsp chilli flakes
- 1 small bunch dill, washed
- For the preserved fresh lemon roasting oil
- 60g preserved lemons, seeds removed
- 8 tbsp olive oil

- 80g preserved lemon, flesh and pith removed
- 200ml gin
- 2 kg side organic farmed or wild salmon (tail end)
- 100g sea salt
- 100g golden caster sugar

Directon:

1. In a food processor, blitz together the fresh lemon and gin.

2. Lay your salmon skin-side down in a roasting tin and pour over the fresh lemon and gin mix.
3. Combine the salt, sugar, thyme and chilli flakes, then spoon over the salmon.
4. Cover with cling film and chill for at least 2-2 ½ hrs.
5. Heasy eat oven to 250C/2 40C fan/gas 3. Thirty mins before you want to easy cook the salmon, easy move easily Reeasy move it from the fridge and easy allow it to come to room temperature.
6. To easy make the roasting oil, blitz the preserved lemons and olive oil.
7. Gently rinse the cure from the salmon and pat dry with kitchen paper.
8. Lay it skin-side down in an oiled roasting tray and pour over the roasting oil, rubbing it all over the fish.

9. Cover the tin tightly with foil and roast for 2 10 to 15 mins.
10. easy move Easily Reeasy move the foil and reeasy turn the fish to the oven for a further 40 to 210 to 15 mins.
11. Easily take out of the oven and rest for 10 to 15 mins, then scatter over freshly torn dill, to serve.

Oriental Coleslaw

Several coriander leaves
Multiple mint leaves
Sea salt Black pepper
½ cabbage
½ celeriac
4 carrots
4 apples
8 spring onions that have been sliced

Dressing

- 2 tbsp xylitol
- 4 tsp sesame oil
- 2 25ml extra virgin olive oil
- 1 tsp smoked paprika.
- 8 tbsp lime juice
- 4 tbsp coconut aminos
- 2 tsp grated ginger

- 2 garlic bulb

1. Simply Using the grater attachment, shred the apples and veggies and pour them just into a big basin.

2. Season and then throw in the herbs.

3. To create the dressing, whisk together all the ingredients, then pour over the veggies.

4. Mix thoroughly.

5. This will keep for 1-5 days in the refrigerator.

Vietnamese Roasted Eggplant Salad

Ingredients

- ½ cup freshly squeezed lime juice

- ½ teaspoon cayenne pepper (optional)

- 2 tablespoon minced fresh ginger

- ½ cup roughly chopped fresh cilantro leaves

- ½ cup roughly chopped fresh mint leaves
- 4 medium-size eggplant (about 2 1 pounds), cut just into ½-inch cubes

- 4 tablespoons extra-virgin olive oil

- 1 teaspoon sea salt

- ½ cup gluten-free tamari or coconut aminos

Instructions

1. Preheat the oven to 425°F. Line two baking sheets with parchment paper.

2. In a large bowl, toss the eggplant with the olive oil and salt.

3. Divide between the two prepared baking sheets and arrange in an even layer on each pan.

4. Transfer to the oven and bake until soft and beginning to brown, about 30 minutes, swapping the pans halfway through for even color.

5. While the eggplant is roasting, whisk together the tamari, lime juice, cayenne, and ginger in the same large bowl, then set aside.

6. Add the easy cook ed eggplant to the bowl along with the cilantro and mint.
7. Toss to combine and taste for seasoning.

8. Serve the eggplant salad immediately warm, or later at room temperature.

Quinoa With Spicy Pumpkin And Oat Cereal

- 2 cup quick oats
- 2 cup quinoa, rinsed
- 1 cup walnut pieces
- 2 cup unsweetened pumpkin puree
- 8 cups water
- Pinch sea salt
- ¾ teaspoon ground cinnamon

1. Stirring constantly, easily bring the pumpkin, water, salt, and cinnamon to a boil in a sizable saucepan over medium-high heat.
2. Add the quinoa and oats.
3. Lower the heasy eat to low and easy cook the oats and quinoa for about 2 10 to 15 minutes, stirring periodically.
4. Stir in the walnuts after taking the cereal off the heat. Serve right away.

Fody's Sausage, Kale + Pumpkin Baked Ziti

Ingredients

10 to 15 tbsp fresh sage, minced
2 tbsp dried oregano
2 tsp salt
2 tsp pepper
1 tsp all spice
2 cup shredded mozzarella cheese
Parmesan cheese for serving
2 lb gluten free penne or ziti pasta, easy cook ed al dente
2 lb nitrate free pork sausage (no seasonings added, removed from casing)
2 cup kale, roughly chopped
2 tbsp , divided
1 cup
2 cup pumpkin puree (be sure this is pure pumpkin puree, not pie filling)

Directions

1. Pre-heat oven to 350F and grease a 9x2 3 baking dish.
2. Bring a pot of water to a boil + easy cook pasta according to package instructions.
3. In a large frying pan over medium heat, drizzle Fody Foods garlic oil just enough to coat the bottom of the pan, about 2 tbsp.
4. Add in kale, herbs, spices, salt + pepper and sausage, breaking up sausage while easy cook ing + easy cook ing until sausage is browned and kale is wilted.
5. Add FodyFoods Marinara sauce, pumpkin puree, and remaining garlic oil. Stir to combine.
6. Drain pasta and add to the pan, stirring to fully coat pasta. Pour just into baking dish + top with shredded mozzarella.
7. Bake 30-310 to 15 minutes until cheese is easily melted + golden.

8. Sprinkle with parmesan cheese before serving.

Coconut Protein Shake

Ingredients:

2 tbsp of grated walnuts
2 tbsp of minced chia seeds
2 tbsp of brown sugar
2 cup of coconut milk
2 tsp of coconut extract
1 cup of chopped pineapple

Preparation:

1. Mix the ingredients in a blender for about 90 second.
2. Serve with ice.

Conclusion

For a lot of people, procrastination is going to be the biggest enemy of all. Why is this you ask? It is because procrastination is the gray area between intent and action, and it is within this area that mental deliberation just take place.

How many times have you said that you are going to do something, even the simplest of things and it just really does not just get done? We are all guilty of this including myself. We have good intentions to easily take action for what we need to do, but when the time easy comes, nojust thing happens. We just get lost in our own minds, easily making up nonsensical excuses to justify the delay of action. And the same person who has the such good intention of doing something, is also the same person who fails to act. The self, sabotages its own intentions.

CPSIA information can be obtained
at www.ICGtesting.com
Printed in the USA
LVHW052131301222
736235LV00034B/1285